Colostrum

Amazing Immune System Enhancer

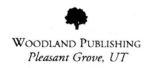

WOODLAND PUBLISHING
Pleasant Grove, UT

Contents

Colostrum: Mother Nature's Immunity Food

THE LAST SEVERAL DECADES have seen the advent of many shifts in the research concerning the immune system of the body. The recent discovery that colostrum carries agents that can positively affect immune function in humans is indeed valuable. Through an impressive body of research, it is evident that colostrum is responsible for the first transmission of immune signals in a newborn, signals that are valuable in shaping the knowledge of the newborn's defense systems. When an infant human (or animal) is born, the immune system is relatively "naive" to the various invaders waiting to break down its defense systems and take over the body. So, as colostrum is the first food that the newborn traditionally takes in, the information that the mother has collected over her lifetime concerning how to effectively fight microbial invaders, cancerous cells, and other toxins is immediately transferred to her newborn. In a time when the infant is especially vulnerable to literally thousands of vicious invaders, Nature has provided a way to aid the infant in the process of building his or her immune system, both quickly and effectively. Of course, colostrum is an essential part of this complex and timely process.

So, when does this process begin exactly? Immediately follow-ing birth, the newborn is generally fed. And the first portion of fluid that comes from the mother is colostrum, an exceedingly nourishing and vital food. For decades, it was thought by experts that colostrum contained only vital nutrients in a nutritional sense; that is, that it contained high levels of protein, fats, vita-mins, etc. (As a side note, because of this, many people, including so-called experts, believed that baby formula could essentially replace a mother's milk.) Of course, most pediatric doctors, nutri-tionists, and scientists now believe that breast-feeding a child is much more beneficial than simply bottle-feeding a child with for-mula.

In addition, we now have discovered that colostrum (and breast milk in general) is much more than a nutrient-rich fluid. Prior to delivering an infant, the expectant mother prepares with-in herself a mix of immune agents that are included almost exclu-sively in the colostrum that the newborn is provided. This mix contains agents that are not species-specific in their function. What this means is that these immunizing agents (sometimes referred to as "growth factor," "immune factor," "suppression factor," "transfer factor" and other names) do not produce an allergic reaction when introduced to a foreign species (or another member of the same species, for that matter). Simply stated then, this means that the specific immune agents produced by a horse are just as effective in chickens or humans as they might be in another horse. Or, for matters dealing with alternative health, and since most colostrum food supplement products contain cow, or bovine colostrum, this means that a cow's specific agents could transfer the valuable immunizing data to a human without pro-voking an allergic response. This exciting development in the world of medicine could have far-reaching implications, especial-ly in the areas of infectious diseases that currently ravage our planet. Some of the more prominent and devastating conditions that could effectively be prevented by use of colostrum and its amazing properties are viral and bacterial infections, parasitic infections, autoimmune disorders, neurological conditions, fungal infections, tissue damage (such as in the intestinal tract), and many others.

Defending the Fort: An Overview of the Body's Immune System

The body uses a myriad of processes, mechanisms and agents to defend itself. All of these make up what is commonly known as the immune system (although there simply is no one thing or system). This section will be a simplified account of how the body defends itself using various processes and components that are generally categorized as the immune system. The body basically uses three interrelated functions—recognition, response, and recall—in making its defense mechanisms effective. First, the body is able to recognize foreign agents within the body; these can include anything from a virus to a toxin from cigarette smoke. Once this foreign agent is recognized, the body enlists the help of a variety of cells and molecules to eliminate or neutralize the invader. Finally, and maybe most importantly, the body is able to remember, or recall, the exact specific—such as mode of action—of the foreign substance so that next time it comes around, it can quickly and effectively deal with it.

To be able to enter the body, the invading organism must first get through physical barriers like the skin and mucous membranes of the nose, throat, and sinuses. These provide an extremely effective barrier to entry by most microorganisms. Intact skin is the most effective barrier; it is compromised when it experiences cuts, scrapes and other wounds. To otherwise gain entry into the body, pathogens must colonize into a formidable number to be able to withstand the various defense cells of the mucous membranes and discharge of mucus by the body to penetrate the mucous membrane. The number of the pathogen must be great enough to withstand the "washing" by saliva, tears, mucous and other fluids, most of which also possess antibacterial and antiviral properties.

If the invading organisms are able to get through the skin and mucous membranes, there are several other immune system barriers waiting. The body's temperature is an effective deterrent to many organisms. For instance, anthrax, a serious condition common to many farm animals, does not affect chickens because of the chickens' high body temperature. Hydrochloric acid, found in the stomach, is also a major barrier to infection. Very few viruses that make it past the mucous membranes of the nose and throat to the stomach can survive the stomach's acid and low pH. Interferon is another of the body's great immunity agents. It is derived from virus infected cells, thereby enabling it to bind with and neutralize nearby virus cells; if there is enough of the interferon, it can neutralize large numbers of the invading virus.

FRONT-LINE DEFENSE: THE BODY'S FIGHTER CELLS

As mentioned before, the body uses agents to effectively defend itself from invading organisms and cells. These are commonly referred to as "fighter" cells. There are two major groups of fighter cells, or phagocytes (any cell that destroys foreign particles) in the immune system: antigen producing cells, called B-lymphocytes, and T-cells, produced by the thymus gland. These antigen producers are supported by other glands in the body, which include the lymph nodes, spleen, the tonsils, appendix and Peyer's patches. One of the most wonderful characteristics of these producers is their capability to overtake the production of antigens that normally would be handled by another "producer" that has for some reason or other become unable to.

Simply stated, the immune system is an extremely complex and multifaceted system that is made up of over a trillion cells. As mentioned before, the immune system performs three very important tasks. First, it has the ability to recognize alien like bacteria, viruses, parasites, and toxins; next, it reacts to each pathogen as an individual invader; and last, once the whole system has come in contact with a pathogen, it remembers the alien and quickly acts upon its possible invasion.

What is extremely interesting in how the body reacts against invading organisms is that it generally doesn't do it the same way every time. The immune system has two separate reactions to invading or foreign agents. The first response involves the production of immunoglobulins, otherwise known as antibodies. This response is called the humoral immune reaction and is targeted against foreign organisms and cells. The second response is cell-mediated immunity (CMI) and, as its name implies, depends on interactions between the many forms of immune system cells (lymphocytes). This response is directed mainly against the body's own cells that turn cancerous or become infected. One important note is that many of these invading cells mutate and change their basic structures on a regular basis to avoid being identified by the body's immune cells. That is why we continually experience common colds, flu and other infections.

Colostrum and Immune Function

Communication between cells is entirely essential to a smooth running immune system. To communicate between cells, the system uses hormone-like signal substances, many of which are usually found in colostrum. While researching tuberculosis, Dr. H. Sherwood Lawrence discovered that an immune response could literally be transferred from a donor to a another recipient by injecting that person with an extract of leucocytes. Dr. Lawrence and others figured this extract contained a factor capable of passing on the donor's immunity to the recipient. (Hennen, 1997)

The exact constituents of colostrum have eluded exact identification for many years. To begin with, colostrum extracts have been estimated to contain more than 200 individual compounds that may play a part in this essential communication process.

So, where does colostrum really play a part in all this? For instance, an immature response within the immune system to an infection may take anywhere from ten days to two weeks to completely develop. Colostrum and its specific components can help reduce this delay in reaction time because they include two factors, or functions—inducer/helper functions and a suppressor function. The inducer function helps the body develop a mature response, even in as little time as twenty four hours. However, an overactive immune response to ever-present agents such as pollens or even the body's own cells certainly is not healthy. This is where the suppression factor comes in, to help control hyperreactive responses that are commonly manifested as allergies and autoimmune diseases. All of this helps keep the immune system and the body's overall health balanced.

Like we discussed earlier, an infant's first food is usually the mother's milk, which initially is comprised of nutrient-rich colostrum. Additionally, colostrum contains valuable components that help the immune system communicate or pass on information between cells. Unlike immunoglobulins, there are other agents that are not species-specific. In other words, there are agents that come from one species that are equally effective in another species. This also means that these agents generally do not cause allergies.

Conditions for Which Colostrum and Its Derivatives Can be Used

COLOSTRUM AND HERPES

Herpes is commonly found in today's world, and is a disease that manifests itself in recurrent outbreaks, characterized by sores and other skin lesions. In one recent study concerning herpes and colostrum agents, a group of thirty-seven patients was tested to see how they would respond to treatment. The results were very promising. Sixty-two percent showed marked improvement in their condition by either a decrease of the frequency of outbreaks and/or a shortening of the duration of any experienced outbreak. These results are impressive for a couple of reasons. To put this in the proper perspective, this group was suffering an average of twelve outbreaks every year. After therapy with the colostrum agents, however, the number of relapses was cut by nearly 75 percent—or 3.5 per year. Even the group that had the most resistant conditions experienced a 50 percent success rate.

Another study delivered an equally impressive outcome. In this study, forty-four patients suffering from both genital labial herpes were orally treated with bovine colostrum agents. These patients recorded their average times in between suffering symptoms. Previous to treatment with colostrum agents, their average symptom-free time was 49 days. After treatment, their symptom-free time increased nearly three-fold, to 140 days.

Other studies back up these findings. Studies from China, Europe and elsewhere have shown colostrum and its specific immune-enhancing agents to have great success in treating the various forms of herpes. These findings are especially amazing when considering how difficult and marginally successful conventional medicine is in treating herpes.

COLOSTRUM AND HEPATITIS

It has been noted that the use of agents withing colostrum that are specifically programmed to fight the hepatitis viruses has a very protective role in even preventing the onset of hepatitis. Additionally, research has shown that the use of these agents also is extremely effective in limiting the recurrence of flare-ups or symptoms. One such study was especially interesting. In this study, fifty-two cases of chronic, active hepatitis were examined. After the treatment regimen of bovine colostrum agents, symptoms either improved or disappeared in 100 percent of the cases. Even more impressive was the fact that any cold, flu or bouts of fatigue that the subjects were experiencing were virtually eliminated by the treatment.

COLOSTRUM AND CHRONIC FATIGUE SYNDROME

Another puzzling and recently emerged conditions is chronic fatigue syndrome. Chronic fatigue is a syndrome with many and various factors that contribute to its onset. Of course, it is no mystery to most researchers and health professionals that viral infections can play a big role in the development of chronic fatigue syndrome. Because of colostrum's wide range of agents that can act against specific viruses and toxins, and because of the somewhat mysterious causes of CFS, it seems natural that colostrum may be a potent treatment to reverse the syndrome's effects. Other studies back up this notion.In one study, nearly 90 percent of the study's cases experienced significant success. In a 1996 Italian study, 60 percent of the subjects began to experience relief within three to six weeks after beginning treatment. Finally, one study using colostrum agents specific to herpes was used to treat patients with chronic fatigue syndrome. The results were certainly encouraging. Say the researchers concerning what they found, ". . . Treatment significantly improved the clinical manifestations of CFS within weeks. . . . It is concluded that HHV-6 specific TF [a colostrum agent] may be of significant value in controlling HHV-6 [herpes] infection and related illnesses."

As mentioned earlier, because of chronic fatigue's uncertain and various causal factors, a substance such as colostrum, which may contain literally dozens of disease-specific agents, could be the most effective in treatments for the syndrome.

Another study was very impressive in colostrum, and specifically transfer factor's, ability to help reverse recurrent cystitis in women, which is usually caused and/or exacerbated by bacterial infection. The subjects had been treated at least once previously with standard drugs, either antibiotics or anti-inflammatory drugs. The study states:

"Results of conventional treatment of female non-bacterial recurrent cystitis (NBRC) are discouraging. Most patients show an unexpected high incidence of vaginal candidiasis, while their cell mediated immunity to Herpes simplex viruses (HSV) and Candida antigens seems impaired, and it is known that the persistence of mucocutaneous chronic candidiasis is mainly due to a selective defect of CMI to Candida antigens. Twenty nine women suffering of NBRC, and in whom previous treatment with antibiotics and non-steroid anti-inflammatory drugs was unsuccessful, underwent oral transfer factor (TF) therapy [transfer factor is one of the many immune agents found in colostrum]. TF specific to Candida and/or to HSV was administered bi-weekly for the first 2 weeks, and then once a week for the following 6 months. No side effects were observed during treatment. . . . It, thus, seems that specific TF may be capable of controlling NBRC and alleviate the symptoms." (DeVinci, 1996)

So, from the researchers own words, specific colostrum agents could be very effective in relieving conditions involving recurrent cystitis, a very painful and annoying condition.

Still another study yielded exciting results concerning colostrum and general viral infections, resulting in herpes, cystitis, candidiasis, uveitis and other conditions. The study's researchers state:

". . . 153 patients suffering from recurrent pathologies, i.e. viral infections (keratitis, keratouveitis, genital and labial herpes) uveitis, cystitis, and candidiasis were treated with in vitro produced transfer factor (TF) [an agent specific to colostrum] specific for HSV-1/2, CMV and Candida albicans. . . . TF administration also significantly increased the soluble HLA class I antigens level in 40 patients studied to this effect." (Pizza, G. 1996)

In other words, there was a noticeable rise in the production of the body's own immune antigens in a sizeable portion of the study's subjects.

COLOSTRUM AND CANDIDIASIS

Because colostrum and its immune agents are effective in helping the body combat various types of invading pathogens, it is also believed that it can help fight conditions like chronic candidiasis. One such study demonstrates that indeed colostrum (and its specific agents) could be effective in relieving and reversing the condition of Candida overgrowth. The researchers state:

"Fifteen patients suffering from chronic mucocutaneous candidiasis were treated with an in vitro produced TF [transfer factor, an agent derived from colostrum] specific for Candida albicans antigens. Clinical observations were encouraging: all but one patient experienced significant improvement during treatment with specific TF. These data confirm that orally administered specific TF, extracted from induced lymphoblastoid cell-lines, increases the incidence of reactivity against Candida antigens." (Masi, 1996)

COLOSTRUM AND CANCER

Cancer is certainly a scary and menacing prospect. While millions and millions of dollars have been pumped into research to find a "cure," many health professionals are pushing for research into nutritional and other preventive measures to fight the war against cancer. Colostrum and its various agents are a promising prospect in the research to both prevent the onset of and fight the development of cancer.

There are a number of studies that investigate the role that colostrum derivatives can have in fighting various forms of cancer. The authors of one recent study state:

"As conventional treatments are unsuccessful, the survival rate of stage D3 prostate cancer patients is poor. Reports have suggested the existence of humoral and cell-mediated immunity (CMI) against prostate cancer tumor-associated antigens (TAA). These observations prompted us to treat stage D3 prostate cancer patients with an in vitro produced transfer factor (TF) [a derivative of colostrum] able to transfer, in vitro and in vivo, CMI against bladder and prostate TAA. Fifty patients entered this study and received one intramuscular injection of 2-5 units of specific TF monthly. Follow-up, ranging from 1 to 9 years, showed that complete remission was achieved in 2 patients, partial remission in 6, and no progression of metastatic disease in 14. The median survival was 126 weeks, higher than the survival rates reported in the literature for patients of the same stage." (Pizza, G, 1996: 123-32)

Another study, which involved patients suffering from lung cancer, showed that colostrum and its immune-enhancing agents can be effective in treating various forms of cancer. The study, which ran for one year, involved 99 lung cancer patients. The researchers state, "The rationale for using transfer factor (an agent specific to colostrum) in lung cancer patients is that the possibility of improving their cell-mediated immunity to tumor associated antigens (TAA) may improve their survival" (Pilotti, 1996).

The results of this study, much like many others involving the use of colostrum and its individual constituents, had great results. The researchers state, "The survival rates of the TF treated group appear significantly improved both for patients in stages 3a and 3b, and patients with histological subtype 'large cell carcinoma.' The results of this study suggest that the administration of TF to NSCLC resected patients may improve survival."

Though these studies suggest that colostrum and its various constituents can be used to treat cancer, it is probably in an immune-enhancing role that they are most valuable. For instance, with conventional radiation treatment, there are usually strong and adverse side effects, including nausea, weight loss, extreme fatigue, etc. The side effects experienced after radiation may be due to the toxicity of the treatment combined with the vast accumulation of sick and dying cells, which the body's own systems would normally deal with. There are a number of studies that show that when given treatments of colostrum agents, these side effects are significantly reduced. This is probably due to the ability of colostrum and its specific compounds to promote immune function in a body where immune function has been greatly reduced by either radiation or chemotherapy.

Other Conditions for Which Colostrum Can Be Used

Since the pioneering research concerning colostrum and the various agents that make up its remarkable immune-enhancing abilities has been conducted, it has long been postulated that treatment with these agents could be a promising treatment for the varied autoimmune conditions that afflict many today.

TYPE I DIABETES: Diabetes is one of the world's most widespread and debilitating of disorder. In addition, Type I diabetes is increasingly being associated with dysfunction of the immune system. There is research showing that colostrum and its specific compounds may have a reversing effect on diabetes. In one trial, colostrum agents were studied in an experimentally induced diabetic condition. The authors of the study theorize that both the inducing and suppressing agents found in colostrum could be involved in the reversing effects on diabetes. Even more encouraging are the results because of the long-lasting effects seen in the study.

INTESTINAL INJURY: Another area in which colostrum has been shown to be an effective healing agent is in the intestinal system. Digestion, stress, and dysfunction can all injure the various parts of this system, including the intestinal walls. But research is now indicating that colostrum and its various constituents can play a vital role in tissue regeneration within the intestinal gut.

One such study reiterates these findings. It is widely known among doctors and health professionals that man drugs, including NSAIDS (which stands for non-steroidal anti-inflammatory drugs) can cause harm to gastrointestinal system. The research team determined to see if colostrum and its growth factors could have a preventive and/or healing effect on injury to the gut. The results were certainly promising. Say the researchers in their conclusion as to colostrum's healing benefits, "Bovine colostrum could provide a novel, inexpensive approach for the prevention and treatment of the injurious effects of NSAIDs on the gut and may also be of value for the treatment of other ulcerative conditions of the bowel" (Playford, 1999).

AUTISM: Put in simple terms, autism is an extremely puzzling and mysterious condition. Like so many other disorders of the neurological and/or immune systems, autism may have many and varying causes. Researchers have determined that one factor that could play a major role in the development of autism is that of viral-caused congenital rubella. In these cases, it's almost as if there is a back-and-forth fight between the body's immune system (often ill-equipped) and the rubella. Of course, it is commonly accepted among researchers that children with autism generally have depressed immune states.

However, research involving colostrum-derived agents shows that autism can be reversed to the extent that a child may be able to return to mainstream school and social activities. The study, which involved twenty-two truly autistic children, revealed that twenty-one of the patients responded to treatment with colostrum-derived agents. And of these twenty-one, ten were able to return to mainstream school and social activities. Particularly disturbing was the finding that of these children, nearly 70 percent (fifteen) began developing symptoms of autism within one week of receiving immunizations for either the measles, mumps, or rubella. The researchers involved in this study state that autism is probably an adverse reaction to a live virus vaccine in an individual whose immune system is not yet mature enough to handle it.

RHEUMATOID ARTHRITIS (RA): Rheumatoid arthritis is another disorder that results from an unexplained attack of the body's own defense systems against itself. A sinister form of this is juvenile rheumatoid arthritis, which attacks children and then remains with them for the remainder of their lives, although the severity can wax and wane. Studies involving colostrum derivatives have demonstrated a good success rate in cases of juvenile rheumatoid arthritis that previously had not responded to even very high dosages of steroids and immunosuppressant drugs.

AIDS: One of the most exciting areas of use for colostrum and its various specific compounds is AIDS. Recently and international symposium on one of colostrum's compounds—transfer factor—was held, and which highlighted the research of various scientists. This groups has had some impressive results in their work with transfer factor and the HIV virus. In fact, some of their research demonstrated favorable results involving transfer factor and Zidovudine, a drug commonly used in AIDS treatment. Some researchers are coming to the realization that the most effective way to treat AIDS should certainly involve the optimal functioning of the individual's immune system. Whether or not a vaccine is produced, it is increasingly more clear that colostrum and its derivatives can provide such a stimulus in this area.

EPSTEIN-BARR: The Epstein-Barr virus is associated with the onset of various symptoms, including extreme fatigue, headaches, and the like. A recent study used colostrum agents with known potency for Epstein-Barr and cytomegalovirus, a dangerous virus responsible for a variety of conditions. The results of this study again showed the remarkable immune-enhancing capabilities of colostrum-derived agents. Two patients showed a total remission of their symptoms, seven demonstrated significant improvement in their symptoms, and five displayed no significant response. In contrast to these findings, a control group that was given a placebo under the same protocol resulted in no real improvement.

What, Why, How?
Commonly Asked Questions
Concerning Colostrum

Q) *Why should an adult need colostrum supplementation?*

A) After going through puberty, our bodies gradually decrease in its production of the immune and growth factors that help combat disease.With the loss of these vital components, we are more susceptible to the aging process, thereby shortening our life expectancy. In addition, colostrum and its various components have the demonstrated ability to ward off bacterial and viral invaders. Finally, colostrum has the ability to stimulate tissue repair (particularly the bowel lining), something that becomes more and more valuable as we age. (See section on colostrum's ability to enhance tissue repair.)

Q) *What should I consider when selecting colostrum?*

A) Colostrum should be collected during the first 24 hours after birth. Additionally, make sure the colostrum is processed in a USDA licensed facility to insure yourself that the USDA guidelines are being followed. In addition, consumers should make sure that products labeled Colostrum are 100% colostrum (not colostrum whey or concentrates of milk whey).

Finally, colostrum mixed with other supplements or herbs and additives may dilute the colostrum concentration and may compromise its benefits .

Q) *Does colostrum interact with other drug or supplements?*

A) Although colostrum has no drug interactions, you may experience side effects from a cleansing or healing crisis, a necessary though somewhat inconvenient and adverse result. However, once the healing crisis is complete, you will feel substantially better in terms of good health.

Also, medications may need to re-evaluated for dose and need by your medical professional.

Q) *Can I take colostrum while pregnant or nursing?*

A) Although generally believed to be very safe for pregnant and nursing mothers, like any supplement or drug, you probably need to ask your medical professional prior to taking colostrum or its specific agents while pregnant.

Q) *Is colostrum supplementation safe for kids?*

A) Colostrum is recommended for children who have not received the mother's breast milk, which would have already provided the benefits that colostrum supplementation can give.

Children with flu, colds, bacterial or viral infections, or children who have been on long- or short-term antibiotics or other drugs are good candidates to receive colostrum supplementation.

Q) *Can colostrum products pass on mad-cow disease?*

A) No case of mad cow disease has been reported in the U.S. to date, and awareness of the disease is extremely high, so it is extremely unlikely to contract mad cow disease from a colostrum product.

Q) *How safe are products containing colostrum and its derivatives?*

A) Overall, supplementation with colostrum and/or products containing derivatives of colostrum has been shown to be very safe. It also has been shown that colostrum is equally effective whether taken by injection or by mouth. In addition, it has been shown that long-term oral administration of colostrum preparations is safe. Finally, because infants and the elderly are the two groups especially at risk for infections, one may wonder how safe colostrum products are for these two groups. Oral administration of colostrum is both a safe, effective and easily accepted form of therapy for these two groups.

Completing the Immune Circle: Complementary Agents to Colostrum

ECHINACEA

Concerning the maintenance and strengthening of the immune system, echinacea is one of the most well-known and respected. The various echinacea species (E. angustifolia, E. purpurea, and E. pallida are the most commonly used) have yielded an impressive array of chemical constituents possessing pharmacological properties. This would suggest that there is some sort of synergistic action between the compounds to achieve the therapeutic benefits. Echinacea's major constituents with therapeutic properties are polysaccharides, flavonoids, caffeic acid derivatives, essential oils, polyacetylenes, and alkylamides. As stated previously, these constituents are responsible for a number of immunostimulatory, anti-inflammatory, antiviral, antibacterial and anticancer properties (Murray, 93).

Echinacea and the Immune System

Echinacea exerts several effects on the immune system. One of these influences what is called the alternate complement pathway, which enhances the movement of white blood cells into the areas of infection. Inulin, one of echinacea's most highly regarded compounds, is thought to be responsible for this. Echinacea is also thought to increase the production of properdin, a serum protein that also enhances the activity of the alternate complement pathway (Murray, 97).

Echinacea also affects many of the immune systems various cells responsible for retarding viral and bacterial infection. For instance, it is known to stimulate the activity of the body's T-cells, or lymphocytes, resulting in more production of interferon. These T-cells are also responsible for what is called "cell-mediated immunity." Dr. Michael Murray, a well-respected naturopathic physician, explains, "Cell-mediated immunity refers to immune mechanisms not controlled or mediated by antibodies. Cell-mediated immunity is extremely important in providing resistance to infection by moldlike bacteria, yeast, fungi, parasites, and viruses" (98).

Echinacea's Antiviral Properties

It is known that the aerial portion of *E. purpurea*, as well as extracts of its root, is effective in warding off viruses. Studies have demonstrated that echinacea inhibits various types of viruses, including the influenza (flu), herpes and vesicular stomatitis virus (Murray, 99). How does echinacea work when fighting the onset of virus infection? It is known to block virus receptors on the cell surface, but its most significant action may be that of inhibiting the viruses production of hyaluronidase, the enzyme responsible for allowing virus cells to spread and become more invasive. Echinacea's ability to restrict hyaluronidase production is probably its most impressive antiviral capability.

Echinacea is also able to "kill" viruses indirectly by encouraging the production and release of interferon, the substance capable of blocking the transcription of viral RNA (and thereby blocking its reproduction).

VITAMIN C

One of the most well-known nutrients for promoting basic immune functions is vitamin C. For years (largely due to Dr. Linus Pauling's research on the vitamin), its benefits have been known. There is a large body of research that indicates that it is effective in reducing the severity and duration of colds and flu. Additionally, beyond its antiviral and antibacterial properties, vitamin C acts as an immunostimulant. It enhances white blood cell production, increases interferon (a group of proteins released by white blood cells that combat a virus) levels and antibody responses, promotes secretion of thymic hormones, and improves connective tissue.

Of special note is the necessity of vitamin C for elderly individuals. An increase in age usually brings a decrease in immune system function, thereby allowing for greater risk of infection and disease. Studies have shown that supplementation with vitamin C results in significant improvement in immune function in elderly persons.

One of the great things about vitamin C is that it is found abundantly in various fruits and vegetables—this lends to its being consumed in acceptable amounts without having to take supplements. The best food sources include broccoli, sweet peppers, collards, cabbage, spinach, kale, parsley, melons, potatoes, tangerines and Brussels sprouts. Of course, there are many other foods that are excellent sources of vitamin C.

GARLIC

Garlic (*Allium sativum*), whose culinary prowess is extremely well known, is one of the most commonly used medicinal herbs, found throughout the world and having been employed for various therapeutic purposes for thousands of years. It is common in Chinese herbal medicine, ayurvedic medicine, and has recently received much attention from mainstream news media in the U.S. and other Western countries. Recent research indicates that it possesses some powerful capabilities relating to the immune system and the body's ability to fight infection.

So, how does garlic aid the body in fighting viral infection? Like other herbal and natural substances, garlic possesses antiviral and antibacterial capabilities and has been shown repeatedly to stimulate and improve performance by the body's immune systems. First and foremost, garlic has been shown to kill viruses.

Garlic can also protect the body from invading virus cells by enhancing the body's immune functions. For instance, several of garlic's chemical constituents, including allicin and diallyl trisulfide, have been shown in studies to activate the body's natural killer cells and macrophages, increase B-cell activity and increase the production of antibodies (Bergner 109-110). All this equates to improved chances of resisting infection by invading viruses, bacteria, and other dangerous pathogens. The following is a list of the most prominent viruses, bacteria, and other microbes inhibited by garlic: Candida albicans, Cryptosporidium, Escherichia coli, Herpes simplex virus types 1 and 2, human rhinovirus type 2, influenza B, Mycobacterium tuberculosis, Parainfluenza virus type 3, and Streptococcus faecalis (Bergner 101).

GOLDENSEAL

Goldenseal (*Hydrastis canadensis*), which is native to North America, was used extensively by Native American tribes for a wide variety of ailments, including infections. It is currently a favorite among herbalists for its proven therapeutic capabilities. The pharmacological activity of the plant is attributed mainly to three alkaloids: canadine, hydrastine and berberine. There is substantial research to back up these alkaloids' effect on various bacteria and viruses. Berberine, for instance, has demonstrated the ability to inhibit the activity of Staphylococcus spp., Streptococcus, spp., Chlamydia spp., and Salmonella typhi, and is recognized as the plant's most valuable constituent.

Another reason goldenseal is effective in combating invasion of colds and flu is that of its ability to stimulate the immune system. Berberine stimulates the activity of macrophages, one of the body's defense mechanisms directly responsible for destroying invading viruses, bacteria, cancer cells and other "invaders." Berberine has also been shown to enhance blood flow to the spleen, which has several responsibilities in aiding the body's immune responses (Murray, Pizzorno 67).

PAU D'ARCO

Pau d'arco (*Tabebuia avellanedae*), also known as "taheebo" and "lapacho," is another herbal supplement known for its powerful antiviral, antibiotic and immune system enhancing capabilities. Lapachol, beta-lapachone, hydroxynapthoquinone and other constituents have been shown to actively inhibit the activity of several viruses, including both herpes viruses (I and II), the influenza viruses, polioviruses and vesicular stomatitis virus. (Linhares and De Santana, Lagrota, et al., and Selway). In The Healing Power of Herbs, Dr. Michael Murray says concerning beta-lapachone's antiviral activity: "Studies of beta-lapachone's antiviral activity have offered insights into the mechanism of this powerful quinone. In experiments with viruses, beta-lapachone demonstrated its ability to inhibit certain key viral enzymes, such as DNA and RNA polymerases, and retrovirus reverse transcriptase. These actions have great significance in the possible treatment of acquired immunodeficiency syndrome (AIDS), Epstein-Barr virus, and other viral infections" (223).

ASTRAGALUS

Astragalus (*Astragalus membranaceus*) is extremely popular in Chinese herbal medicine, where it is employed for a wide variety of ailments. It is recognized by Chinese herbalists as an immune system enhancer. But its reputation is not limited to just folk use. There have been clinical trials conducted, most of them in China, that have demonstrated that both the severity and length of the common cold are reduced by application of astragalus (Chang, But 1041-46).

BETA CAROTENE (VITAMIN A)

Vitamin A (and its precursor beta carotene) has long been known to be effective against infectious diseases, including the common cold and the various flu strains. It has antiviral and antibacterial capabilities. A deficiency of vitamin A can manifest itself through increased infection by cold/flu viruses.

Diet, Nutrition, Exercise and Lifestyle Factors in Maintaining a Healthy Immune System

EAT HEALTHFUL FOODS

Eating right will not only help prevent viral and bacterial infections, but will also help promote overall good health. Healthful eating habits encourage healthy cell and tissue reproduction, maintain strong bone and tissues, provide the necessary nutrients for the immune system to operate at top levels, and allow the body to run efficiently and avoid unnecessary stress. Ensure that your diet follows the guidelines given by the FDA , namely the "Food Pyramid." This pyramid outlines the different food groups and the approximate servings one should eat daily to encourage good levels of health.

It is important to remember that there are several factors that determine how one should eat. Age is one of these. For example, most young to middle age adults should consume about 2,000 calories. This number decreases, however, once you are over fifty. The older you are, the "smarter" you must eat. Metabolism slows with age, as does the body's ability to effectively utilize nutrients. Studies show that as one's age increases, so does their risk of contracting more severe strains of infectious diseases.

Probably one of the most sound pieces of advice when determining what and how to eat is that of eating "whole" foods; that is, foods that are in their basic, or natural, state. These would include fresh fruits and vegetables, nuts, and whole grains. Of course, dishes including any of these would generally be considered healthful. Whole foods contain "phytonutrients," compounds such as flavonoids, essential fatty acids, and antioxidants that protect the body and provide the necessary elements for optimal function. As foods are broken down more and more (e.g., processed, cooked, synthesized), their most valuable components are often lost. One cannot overestimate the importance of a healthful diet in not only preventing the onset of minor and major diseases, but of achieving overall good health.

DRINK PLENTY OF FLUIDS

Because nearly seventy-five percent of the body is water, and because water is necessary for most of the body's defense functions, it is very important to keep the body's fluid level's at optimum levels. A typical adult needs at least eight 8-ounce glasses of water or clear liquids a day. Schedule breaks throughout your day to make sure you receive adequate fluids.

EXERCISE

Exercise is essential for overall good health. Aerobic exercise is especially beneficial; it speeds up the heart to pump larger quantities of blood; makes you breathe heavier and faster to aid in the oxygen transfer from the lungs to the cardiovascular system; and forces your body to flush out toxins through sweat once the body's temperature rises. Eventually, aerobic exercise forces the body's cells to use larger amounts of the blood's oxygen, making those body tissues more healthy and able to defend themselves.

Exercise also helps the body by relieving stress; it gets rid of excess adrenaline, triggers the release of endorphins, which helps relieve depression, and strengthens muscles, bones and body tissues. Studies also show that the body's immune system is directly aided by exercise because of the increased release of the body's virus-killing cells.

Basically, exercise is very beneficial for the body's overall health, and can help prevent infection by any virus, bacteria or other invading pathogen. It doesn't really matter what kind of exercise you do; the important thing is that you do it.

AVOID SMOKING

Smoking does several things to promote the onset of various diseases. Smoking dries the cilia in the mucous membranes, paralyzing them in their ability to trap and sweep out viruses and other invaders. Smoking also introduces an overload of toxins to the mucous membranes, making it nearly impossible for the cilia that aren't disabled to get rid of these toxins and any other pathogens. There is an overwhelming mountain of evidence pointing to a direct link between smoking and all forms of respiratory ailments.

AVOID CONSUMING ALCOHOL

Alcohol is a depressant that slows body responses to the environment, including that of eliminating invading viruses, bacteria, parasites, and other microbes. As most people know, heavy alcohol consumption destroys the liver, one the main organs involved in cleaning and filtering the body of unwanted toxins. Alcohol also depletes mineral and vitamin stores and is dehydrating to the body, further diminishing the body's ability to battle the onset of infectious diseases.

GET PLENTY OF REST

The importance of sleep and rest in optimizing the body's ability to fight infection cannot be overemphasized. Numerous studies show that Americans in general do not get enough good quality sleep. Sleep is the time the body is at its best in cleaning the body of unwanted materials, repairing damaged cells, supplying nutrients and essentially revitalizing the body.

REDUCE STRESS

Stress is one of the most common factors contributing to the onset of infectious diseases and other ailments. While stress is a natural part of life, it can sometimes overwhelm a person. There is much research indicating that effective stress management not only helps prevent the onset of various diseases, but also shortens their duration. Identifying and coping with sources of stress can certainly help maintain a healthy immune system.

Summary

Recent advances in medicine have brought hope to researchers and the public alike for a brighter future in health care. One of these advances are the discoveries surrounding the use of colostrum and its derivatives in the fight against infectious diseases and the effort to boost immune function.

The following is a summary of some of more prominent conditions for which colostrum can be used to treat:

- chicken pox
- common cold
- rheumatoid arthritis
- bronchitis
- hepatitis
- HIV
- cytomegalovirus
- cystitis
- urinary tract infections
- tuberculosis
- pneumonia
- lupus
- scleroderma
- measles
- flu
- respiratory tract infections
- mononucleosis
- AIDS
- herpes
- Epstein-Barr
- candidiasis
- salmonella
- mycobacterium infections
- parasitic infections
- fibromyalgia
- chronic fatigue syndrome

Bibliography

Ablashi DV, et al., "Use of anti HHV-6 transfer factor for the treatment of two patients with chronic fatigue syndrome (CFS). Two case reports." Biotherapy 1996;9(1-3):81-6.

Bergner, Paul. The Healing Power of Garlic. Rocklin, California: Prima Publishing, 1996.

Burton Goldberg Group. Alternative Medicine: The Definitive Guide. Fife, Washington: Future Medicine Publishing, 1997.

Bystron J, Cech K, Pekarek J, Jilkova J. "Effect of anti-herpes specific Transfer Factor." Biotherapy 1996, 9(1-3), 73-5.

Bystron J, et al., "Personal experience with treatment of recurrent herpes infections using combined nonspecific immunostimulation." Cas Lek Cesk 1992, 131(5), 137-41.

Chang, H.M. and But, P.P.H. Pharmacology and Applications of Chinese Materia Medica, vol. 2. World Scientific Publishing, Teaneck, NJ: 1987, 1041-46.

De Vinci C., et al., "Use of transfer factor for the treatment of recurrent non-bacterial female cystitis (NBRC): a preliminary report." Biotherapy 1996; 9(1-3):133-8.

De Vinci C. et al., "Lessons from a pilot study of transfer factor in chronic fatigue syndrome." Biotherapy 1996;9(1-3):87-90.

Kirkpatrick CH, "Activities and characteristics of transfer factors." Biotherapy 1996;9(1-3):13-6.

Ferrer-Argote VE, et al. "Successful treatment of severe complicated measles with non-specific Transfer Factor." In Vivo 1994, 8(4), 555-7.

Fudenberg HH, Pizza G. "Transfer Factor 1993: New frontiers." Progress in Drug Res. 1994 42, 309-400.

Fudenberg HH, Fudenberg HH. "Transfer Factor: Past, Present and Future." Ann Rev Pharm Tox 1989, 475-516.

Jiang G, Yi Y, Jiang G. "Preparation of hepatitis B-specific immune Transfer Factor and immune RNA as vaccine for hepatitis." Pat. Number 1098315 (1995-02-08). CAS 123:110148.

Jiang G, Yi B, Jiang G. "Compositions containing immunoribonucleic acids and immune Transfer Factors for controlling hepatitis A as well as hepatitis 1B." Pat. Number 1098289 (1995-02-08). CAS 123:123162.

Lagrota, M., et al. "Antiviral Activity of Lapachol." Review of Microbiology 14 (1983): 21-26.

Lawrence HS, Borkowsky W. "Transfer Factor—current status and future prospects." Biotherapy 1996, 9(1-3),,1-5.

Levine, HH. "The use of Transfer Factors in chronic fatigue syndrome: prospects and problems." Biotherapy 1996, 9(1-3), 87-90.

Lieberman, Shari, PhD, Nancy Bruning. The Real Vitamin and Mineral Book. Garden City Park, New York: Avery Publishing Group, 1997.

Linhares, M. and De Santana C.F. "Estudo sobre of efeito de substancias antibioticas obtidas de Streptomyces e vegetais superiores sobre o herpevirus hominis. Revista Instituto Antibioticos, Recife 15 (1975): 25-32.

Masi M. et al., "Transfer factor in chronic mucocutaneous candidiasis." Biotherapy 1996;9(1-3):97-103.

Meduri R, et al., "Efficacy of transfer factor in treating patients with recurrent ocular herpes infections." Biotherapy 1996;9(1-3):61-6.

Murray, Michael T. The Healing Power of Herbs. Rocklin, Ca.: Prima, 1995.

Murray, Michael, N.D., and Joseph Pizzorno, N.D. Encyclopedia of Natural Medicine. Rocklin, California: Prima Publishing, 1991.

Pekarek J, et al. "The clinical use of specific Transfer Factors." Recent Advances in Transfer Factor and Dailyzable Leucocyte Extracts. Maruzen Co, Ltd: Tokyo, Japan. 1992: 256-63.

Pilotti V. et al., "Transfer factor as an adjuvant to non-small cell lung cancer (NSCLC) therapy." Biotherapy 1996;9(1-3):117-21.

Pizza G, et al., "Transfer Factor prevents relapses in herpes keratitis patients: a pilot study." Biotherapy 1994, 8(1), 63-8.

Pizza G., et al., "In vitro studies during long-term oral administration of specific transfer factor." Biotherapy 1996; 9(1-3):175-85.

Pizza G. et al., "A preliminary report on the use of transfer factor for treating stage D3 hormone-unresponsive metastatic prostate cancer." Biotherapy 1996;9(1-3):123-32.

Playford RJ, et al., "Bovine colostrum is a health food supplement which prevents NSAID induced gut damage." Gut 1999 May; 44(5):653-658.

Raise E, et al. "Preliminary results in HIV-1-infected patients treated with Transfer Factor (TF) and zidovudine (ZDV)." Biotherapy 1996, 9(1-3), 49-54.

Schoneberger, D. "The Influence of Immune-Stimulating Effects of Pressed Juice from Echinacea purpurea on the Course and Severity of Colds." Forum of Immunology (8)1992: 2-12.

Selway, J. "Antiviral Activity of Flavones and Flavins." In: Plant Flavonoids in Biology and Medicine: Biochemical, Pharmacological, and Structure-Activity Relationships. New York: Alan R. Liss, 1986: 521-536.

Transfer Factor in the Era of AIDS. Proceedings of the Xth International Symposium on Transfer Factor. Bologna, Italy, 22-24 June 1995. Biotherapy 1996, 9(1-3), 1-185.

Wilson GB, Paddock GV. "Process for obtaining Transfer Factor from colostrum Transfer Factor so obtained and use thereof." Patent Number US4816563 Patent Date 1989-03-28.

Wilson GB, Fudenberg HH. "Use of In Vitro Assay Techniques to Measure Parameters Related to Clinical Applications of Transfer Factor Therapy." US Patent 4610878. Sept. 9, 1986.

Zhang GS, et al., "Evaluation of the effects of acute hepatitis B treated with specific placenta Transfer Factor." Recent Advances in Transfer Factor and Dialyzable Leucocyte Extracts. Maruzen Co, Ltd: Tokyo, Japan. 1992: 217-21.

Zhang, Guangshu. "Method for preparation of anti-b-hepatitis placental Transfer Factor." Pat. Number 1089843 (1994-07-27). CAS 122:170149.